Usui Reiki Level 3

A COMPLETE GUIDE TO THE HOLISTIC HEALING MODALITY

USUI REIKI - MASTER LEVEL

Djamel Boucly

Authors Disclaimer

Although Reiki offers a variety of benefits and is practiced all over the world today, the material in this manual should not be considered to override any diagnosis made by a Qualified Doctor or Specialist. But, it can be considered as an additional form of treatment. The author cannot accept any responsibility for any illness arising out of the failure of the reader and/or student, to seek medical advice from a Qualified Doctor or Specialist.

Important note to the Student/Reader

The purpose of this manual is to offer the reader insight to the teachings and disciplines associated with Third Degree Usui Reiki.

The information in this manual has been derived from the traditional teachings of Dr. Mikao Usui and does not contain any of the Authors personal beliefs and or practices.

In order to use this manual to heal yourself or others, you must first receive the necessary Reiki attunements from a qualified Reiki Master.

Table of Contents

Usui Reiki Master Level 1
Reiki Lineage 7
Welcome to Reiki Master Level 9
   Definition of a Reiki Master 9
   What does it mean to be a Reiki Master 11
   Reiki Master Symbols 11
   Additional uses for Dai Ko Myo 13
Definitions of Tibetan Buddhist Symbols 21
   Sei He Ki 23
   Raku 26
Healing Attunement 29
   How to do a Healing Attunement 29
   Student Reiki Attunements 32
Distant Attunement 45
   How to Perform a Distant Attunement 45
   Self-Attunements 46
   Self-Attunement Using a Ki Ball 47
Advanced Reiki Techniques 51
   How to Perform Psychic Surgery 54
Reiju 63
   Giving a Reiju Empowerment 66
Brain Balancing 71
   How to do Brain Balancing 72
Reiki Crystal Grids 75

Crystal cleansing methods: 76
　　Preparing your Reiki Crystal Grid 76
　　Charging the Grid 79

Teaching Reiki 81
　　Ethics 81
　　Preparing to Teach 82
　　Points to Consider 83
　　Basic Class Outline - Reiki Level 1 87
　　Basic Class Outline - Reiki Level 2 88
　　Basic Class Outline - Reiki Level 3 89

Additional Techniques and Attunements 93
　　Non-Traditional 93
　　Reiki Assessments 97

ATTUNEMENT CHEAT SHEET 101
　　Single Level 1 Attunement 101
　　Combined Level 1 Attunement 103
　　Level 2 Attunement 106
　　Level 3 Attunement 108
　　Healing Attunement 110

Conclusion 113
　　Final Thoughts 114

Becoming a Reiki Master 117

Interesting References 125
　　Books Available Online 126
　　Interesting Reads to Guide You on Your Journey 129

Introduction

Reiki Lineage

If you are in the process of completing your reiki studies, or you have researched reiki on the internet, then you probably would have come across the term "Reiki Lineage". This can be described as a reiki "family tree".

Reiki Lineage is a list of Reiki Masters/Teachers, which starts with the person that taught you reiki and goes back per teacher, to the original founder of reiki Dr. Mikao Usui.

The ideal is to be part of a strong lineage which reveals an unbroken line (of teachers) stretching back directly to Dr. Mikao Usui, the founder of reiki. Reiki Lineage is very important in European Countries.

However, an important factor to consider, is not to place your main focus on the length of your Reiki Lineage, but whether all the teachers in your lineage have remained true to the original teachings of Dr. Mikao Usui.

Once you have completed Usui Reiki Master Level, you too will belong to a lineage of Reiki Masters/Teachers. If you complete your studies with a Reiki Master, your Reiki Master will provide this information to you.

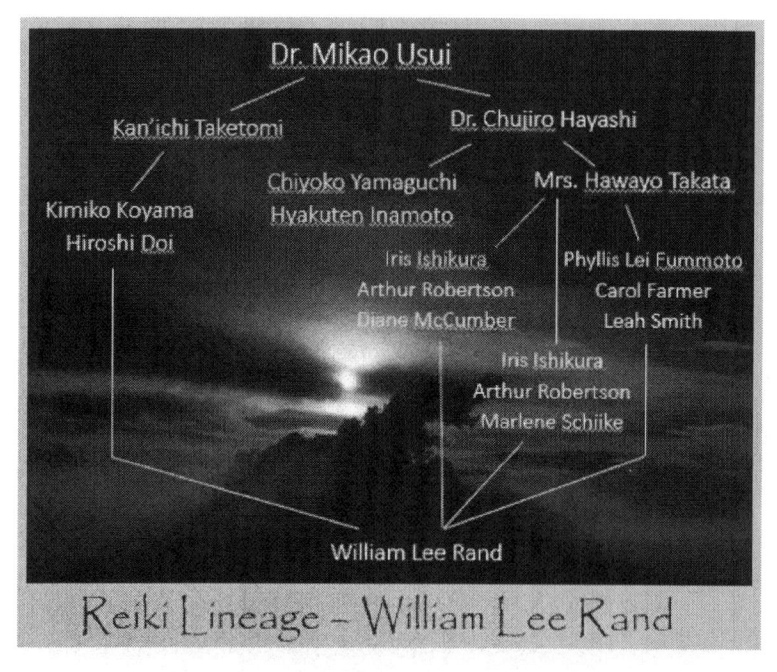

```
                    Dr. Mikao Usui
                   /              \
         Kan'ichi Taketomi      Dr. Chujiro Hayashi
           /                    /              \
                  Chiyoko Yamaguchi    Mrs. Hawayo Takata
    Kimiko Koyama  Hyakuten Inamoto         /    \
    Hiroshi Doi                            /      \
                        Iris Ishikura    Phyllis Lei Fummoto
                        Arthur Robertson  Carol Farmer
                        Diane McCumber    Leah Smith
                                          Iris Ishikura
                                          Arthur Robertson
                                          Marlene Schiike

                         William Lee Rand

         Reiki Lineage – William Lee Rand
```

IMAGE OBTAINED FROM PIXABAY (OCTOBER 2016) AND EDITED/ENHANCED TO ILLUSTRATE "REIKI LINEAGE"

CHAPTER 1

Welcome to Reiki Master Level

Welcome to the third and final module of Usui Reiki training. In Level 1 you were taught basic techniques and the importance of self-healing before you could move on to Level 2, which provided more insight into the practice of Reiki and a guide how to practice Reiki on others.

Level 3 training or Master Level, as it is called will teach you about the master symbol and the attunement process. After completion of Reiki Master Level, you will be able to teach others, do attunements and pass the gift of Reiki on to those who seek inner healing.

Definition of a Reiki Master

Generally "Master" refers to a person who has acquired a complete knowledge in a certain technique and is proficient in their chosen field.

A Reiki Master is seen as someone who has practiced reiki, has a strong knowledge thereof and is proficient in the practice of reiki.

However, there is more to being a Reiki Master than just being proficient in the practice thereof. Reiki becomes part of your life's journey and this is a journey of continued growth and development.

As a Reiki Master one should strive to embrace the essence of reiki and to incorporate the five precepts into ones daily life and dealings with all those in search of healing and love.

Studying Reiki Master Level will qualify you to teach others the practice of Reiki. However, not all students become Reiki Teachers. Some students choose a path of practicing only.

After completion of Usui Reiki Master Level, you may decide for yourself, whether you wish to practice only, or you may take the path of becoming a teacher, or you could decide to do both. Whichever option you choose, your intuition will guide you what to do and your path will be unique to you and your spirit.

Remember that no matter which path you wish to follow, reiki will always be a part of your life and there is nothing more beautiful than passing the knowledge and essence of reiki onto others.

What does it mean to be a Reiki Master

To be a Reiki Master may have different meanings to different Practitioners. But, what you should consider is the following:

It should also mean continued learning and growth, not just mastering a skill or a technique. We learn daily about ourselves and about life. To be a Master means to take that knowledge and share it with whomever crosses your path.

It means to have the purest of intentions, to be sincere and to add compassion and love to all that you do. You should strive to take the knowledge that you have gained and use it to the best of your ability, to assist others on their path to inner healing.

Reiki Master Symbols

In Reiki Level 1 and 2 you learned of the various Reiki Symbols, their meanings and uses and in the Master Level training there is no exception. In this level you will learn of the Usui Master Symbols.

Dai Ko Myo

Usui Master Symbol

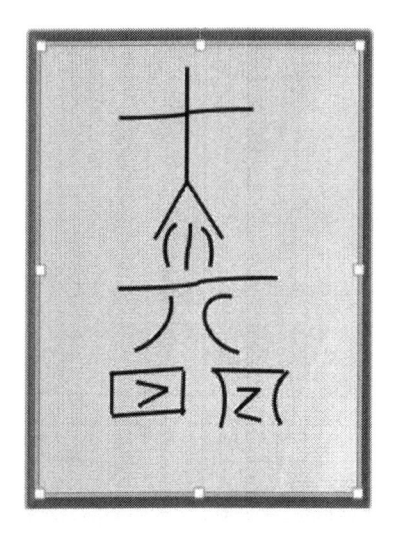

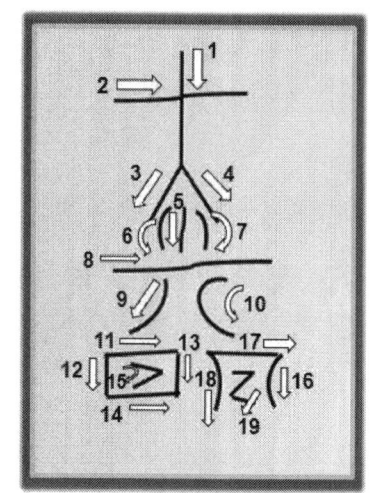

This is the final symbol in traditional Usui Reiki. Pronounced "Die-Coe-Me-Ho". This is a Zen expression of one's own true nature or Buddha-nature. It symbolizes healing of the spirit.

This symbol generally means "Great being of the Universe shine on me, be my friend".

It also means "great shining light".

To further empower the power, mental/emotional and distant symbols, this symbol can be activated first.

The energy associated with the master symbol works on our spiritual body - the highest level of healing.

This master symbol cleanses and heals the spirit. In Karuna Ki it is used to signify the connection of the divine source to compassion.

To activate the energy of this symbol, you have to draw the symbol, visualize it or say its name three times.

Additional uses for Dai Ko Myo

Over and above the "traditional uses of Dai Ko Myo, there are also two exercises which you can do to increase the flow of Ki (energy) through the body and to feel the energy that you are creating. These are as follows:

Focus your mind on the reiki energy until you feel the energy flowing in your palms. Then chant the master symbol's name (silently or out loud) and then say "I establish my divine presence on earth". You can do this as often, or as many times as you wish. Allow yourself the sense the power you are creating.

This exercise can be done twice a day. But, ensure that you back is straight, as posture is important when doing this exercise.

For this exercise you need to find the point in each shoulder blade, located in the bony hollow at the back. Activate reiki energy in your hands, then massage this point (on one shoulder) with your fingertips, in a clockwise motion, for approximately one minute.

Then begin massaging for 300 rotations, using the master symbol. Repeat this process on the opposite shoulder. Complete the full exercise three times. To end the exercise gently make a fist with your right hand and gently tap twenty five times, against your chest (just above the breastbone) and visualize the master symbol whilst you are doing this.

This is a Chi 'Kung exercise which is used for self-healing and it increases the flow of Ki through the body. It also stimulates the hara line, thymus chakra and also improves physical immune function.

This exercise can be done twice a day. But, ensure that you back is straight, as posture is important when doing this exercise.

As people interpret the reiki symbols differently, they have also added their own "new" interpretations of the symbols, over time. You may also come across the symbols drawn in "reverse".

There have also been some new interpretations of the master symbol and you may come across two variations, as below.

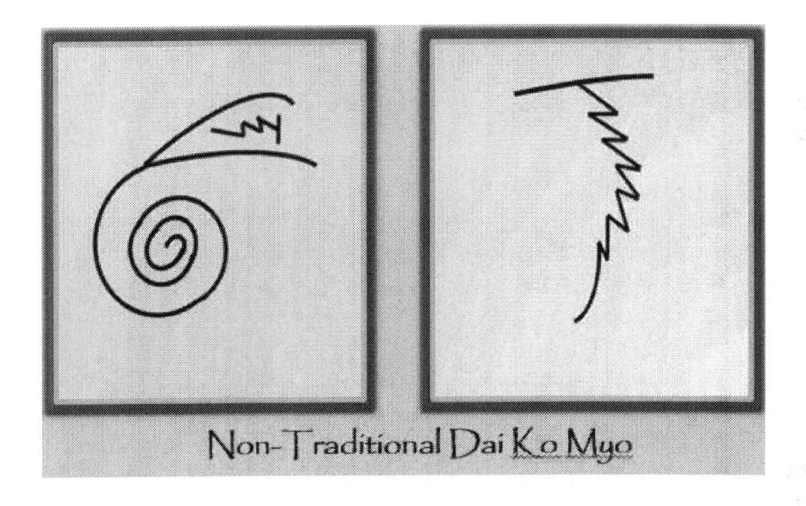

Non-Traditional Dai Ko Myo

Left: Dumo

Right: Tibetan Master Symbol

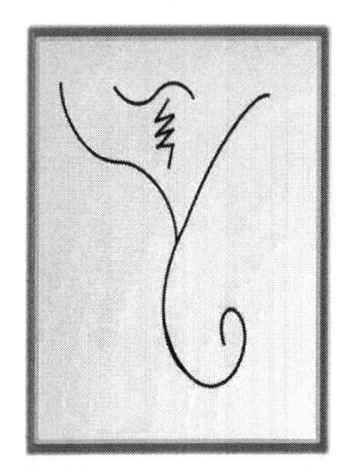

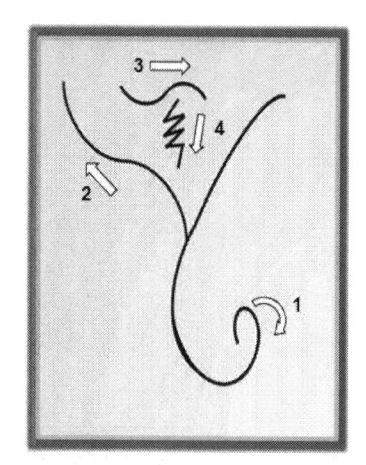

This symbol was not taught in the original Usui Reiki Ryoho. Pronounced "Doo-Moe". Although this was not a traditional symbol, it became so popular, as it is both a beautiful and powerful symbol.

Due to its popularity, it was subsequently included in attunements, as it can be used to activate and anchor the power of the symbol. It symbolizes the connection between the body and the mind.

It enhances spiritual growth, as it connects the body and the mind.

It represents the twirling heat of the Kundalini within.

16

This symbol ignites fire in the root chakra (activates it) and pulls disease and/or negative energy from the body and then releases it.

Left: Fire Serpent

Right: Tibetan Master Symbol

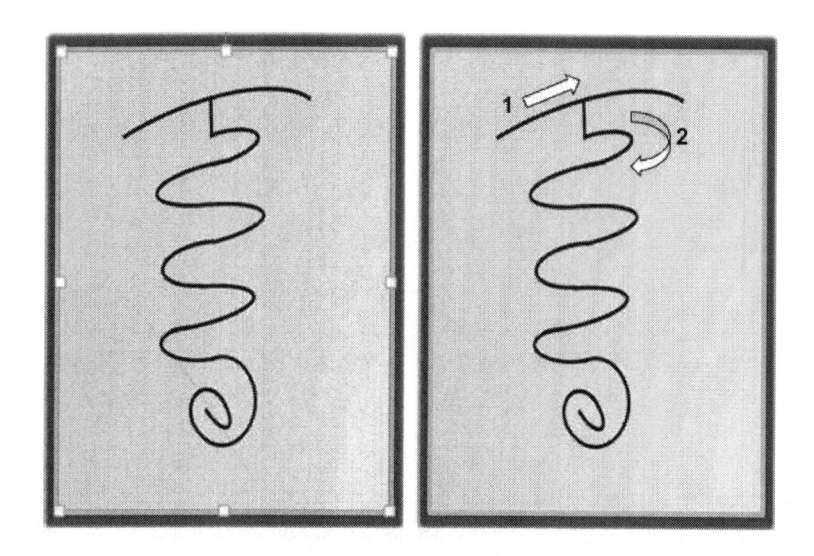

This symbol is also used during the attunement process and is drawn down the student's back. It is used to open and connect all the chakras and enhances balance and harmony.

Using this symbol triggers all the chakras to join together and ultimately allows the attunement energies to enter the student's energy systems more easily.

This symbol signifies the sleeping serpent awakening during the attunement.

This symbol opens the central passage of the Kundalini fire within.

Left: Raku

Right: Tibetan Symbol

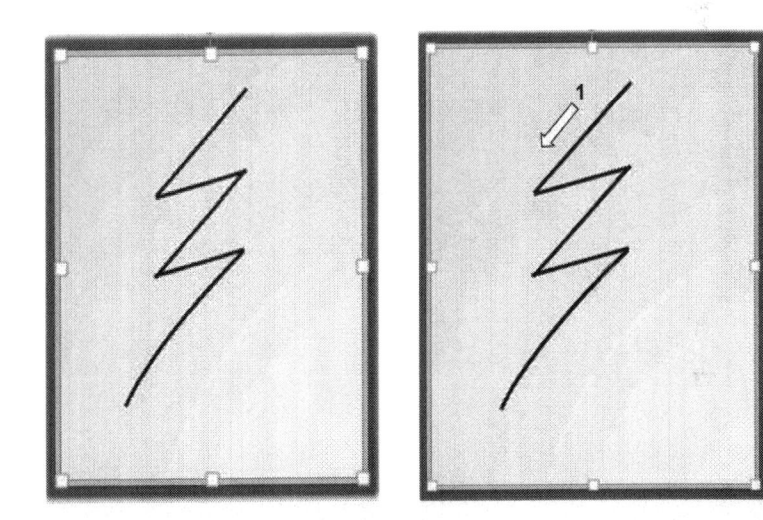

You can use this symbol after every session. Pronounced "Ray-Coo". This symbol grounds and seals the newly awakened reiki energies.

This symbol is known as the "banking of fire" and is used in attunements, not individual healings.

This symbol is used in both Usui and Karuna reiki attunements, or when ending a treatment.

This symbol separates the Master's energy from the initiate/client's.

This symbol can also be used to prevent negative energy from entering into a certain area, i.e. you could use this symbol in the doorway into your office and/or your home.

CHAPTER 2

Definitions of Tibetan Buddhist Symbols

The five reiki symbols represent the five levels of the mind. Together they form the non-duality of mind and object and the absence of ego, which allows one to attain the highest level on the path to enlightenment (referred to as Buddhist Nirvana).

The symbols were not initially intended for healing, but for enlightenment, to help others. To achieve the five levels of wisdom that conclude enlightenment.

Once you achieve enlightenment (Buddhist Nirvana) it releases the being from the wheel of incarnation.

Left: Cho Ku Rei

Right: The Light Switch

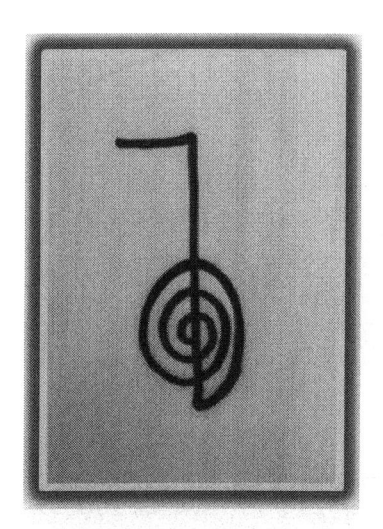

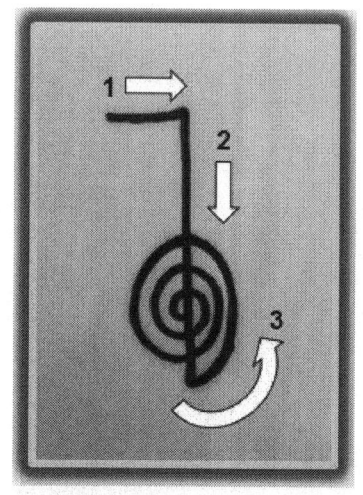

This is the beginning, entry or initiation stage. It places the mandala into the heart. To meditate until there is no difference between the outside world and the meditative state, in order to achieve a state of "emptiness", having no attachment to the earth plane. This is the first experience and the first step.

You may do the following exercise:

Find your quiet "zone" and say the symbols name as a mantra for 108 times and then be aware of what your energy feels like afterwards.

Sei He Ki
Emotional Healing, Purification, Cleansing and Protection

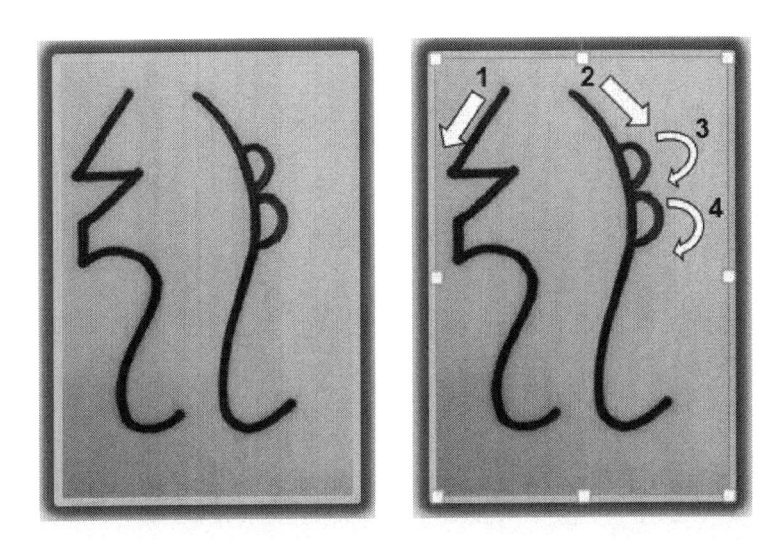

Earth and the human embodiment is considered impure ground. The colour associated with this symbols is yellow (impure), which turns to gold when purified by the fire of wisdom. This is transmutation and purification - the change from impurity to gold.

This is enlightenment, to achieve Buddha status, it is the realization of the emptiness of self. This is where you experience balance between earth and heaven. When you reach Buddha status, the color of your solar plexus will turn to gold.

Hon Sha Ze Sho Nen

Healing past, Present and Future

Distant Healing and Healing Karma

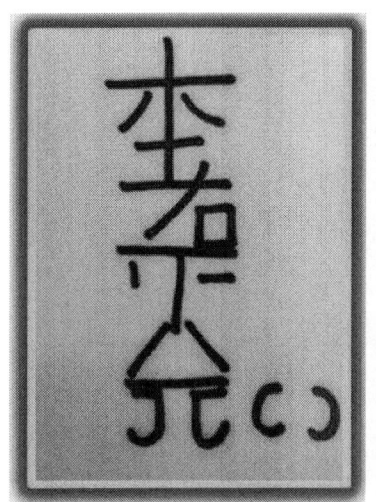

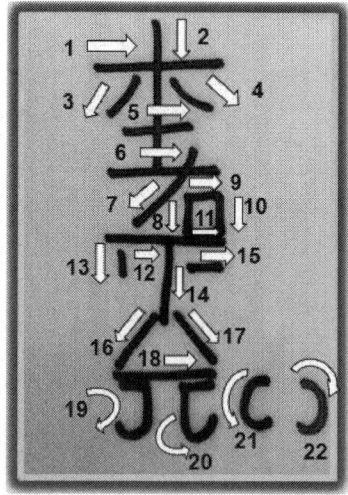

It provides freedom from misconception and karma. (The term Karma refers to the action of the mind). The mind creates time, limitations, space and delusion.

24

Enlightenment is a state where we attain Buddha nature (the Goddess within), a state beyond the mind.

When the mind is in a state of awareness, we are open and we can release. Then we are free from limitations, time, space and delusion. To dispel limitation, will bring us to understand all things.

Left: Dai Ko Myo and Dumo

Right: Healing the Soul

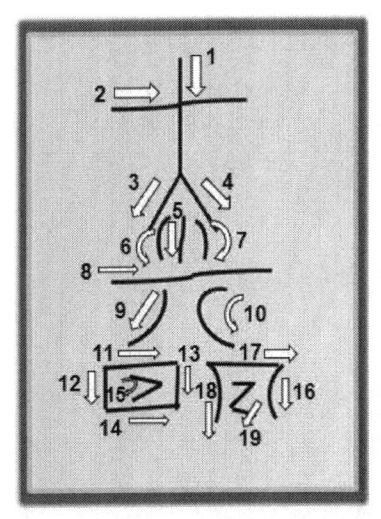

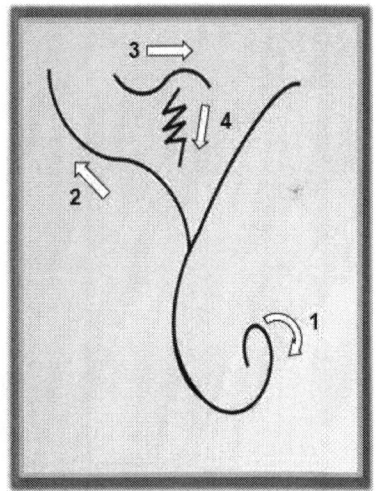

This symbol signifies "The one with the Mahayana heart of giving" or "Temple of the great beaming light". The person who desires enlightenment for the sake of others, will achieve it. One realizes that vast union is the foundation for understanding all things.

This is a state of oneness (the Goddess within). When you become enlightened, you are free from embodiment and suffering. In Buddhism this is regarded as the only real healing. It is the personification of the "mastership - the absolute Buddha nature.

Raku
The Lightning Bolt, Completion and Grounding

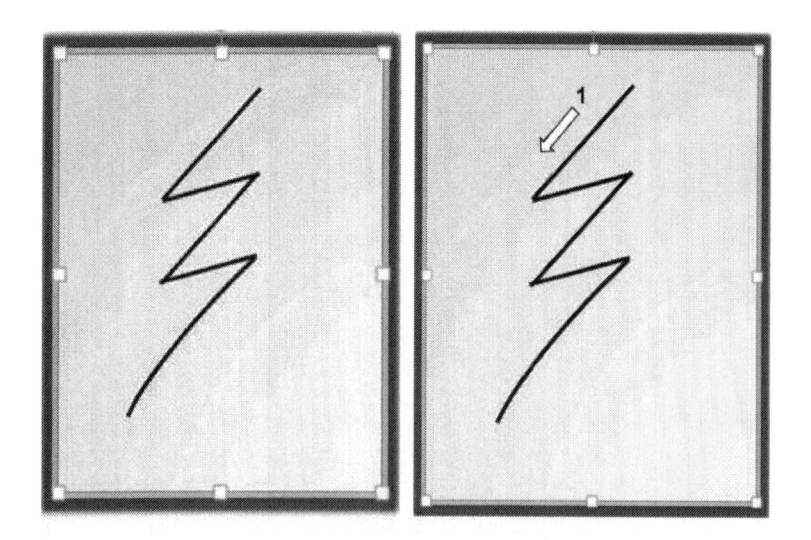

This is achieving lower nirvana (four levels of bliss). It is an emptiness of self and of being. It is the appearance of the image of the Buddha (the Goddess) within oneself. There is enlightenment, freedom and peace.

Freedom from the illusion of the material world, from the body and incarnation. The state of total healing. In reiki this symbol is used from the crown to the feet, to ground the energy and to draw the energy from the universe into the body. To bring spiritual into the "human experience".

However, in Buddhism, it is used from the feet to the crown, in order to take one out of the body. Thus, in Buddhism, this symbol is used for spiritual enlightenment.

CHAPTER 3

Healing Attunement

This technique is similar to the initiation attunement, but it does not open the client to channel reiki. A healing attunement is used to dissolve energetic resistance around the client and to increase the energy available for healing.

It supports the reiki energy, in order that it may work more rapidly and on a deeper level. This is a very effective method to use on clients with more serious concerns.

How to do a Healing Attunement

You may begin the session as you would any "normal" session. Refer to your checklist in the Usui Reiki Level 2 Manual. However, instead of laying down, the client should be seated in an upright position (preferably in a straight backed chair).

Proceed by asking the client the following questions:

To describe the problem which he or she wishes to heal.

If it were in the physical body, where would it be?

If it had a shape, what would it be?

If it had a color, what would it be?

Are you willing to release this blockage?

Then ask the client to close his or her eyes and put their hands in their lap.

- Part One – From the Back

Draw the Fire Serpent from the crown to the root.

Draw Dai Ko Myo, Cho Ku Rei and Hon Sha Ze Sho Nen at the base of the spine.

Place both your hands on the client's head (link and ground).

Draw Dumo above the head (name x 3) and move through the crown to the base of the brain.

Draw Dai Ko Myo above head (name x 3) and move through the crown to the back of the heart.

Repeat heart placement with Cho Ku Rei, Sei He Ki and Hon Sha Ze Sho Nen.

- Part Two – From the Front

Draw Dumo over the crown (name x 3) and move through the 3rd eye down to heart and down to the solar plexus.

Gently tap the crown (x 3) with your fingertips.

Repeat solar plexus placement with Dai Ko Myo, Cho Ku Rei, Sei He Ki and Hon Sha Ze Cho Nen.

Gently blow down toward the solar plexus and up toward the third eye and up to the crown and from the crown back down to the solar plexus in one fluid motion.

Hold the intention (you may use your hands to guide the energy) on the final sweep upward to release all negative energy and move it up and completely out of the energy system.

- Part Three – From the Back

Place both your hands on client's shoulders and visualize a soft pink ball of energy at the heart centre.

Silently and lovingly repeat this affirmation (x 3) – "You are empowered by love, light and wisdom".

Place your dominant hand on the back of the heart centre (other hand remains on the shoulder) and affirm – "I now seal the healing process with love and light" OR "I honour the light and love within you and am grateful to have shared this space in time, in touch, in love with you".

Return your dominant hand to the shoulder silently say this blessing - "We are both blessed by this process".

Disconnect from the energy using Raku.

Then move to the front of the client and have them place their palms on their legs, inhale and on exhalation to open their eyes.

Ask the client to concentrate on the negative shape and to observe changes or its disappearance.

You may now proceed to do a "blockage removal" or a standard reiki session.

Student Reiki Attunements

There are various attunement processes available to use, as follows:

Single Level 1 Attunement

Combined Level 1 Attunement

Level 2 Attunement

Level 3 Attunement

However, most Reiki Masters choose not to do the attunements separately. Most Reiki Masters opt to use the Combined Level 1 Attunement.

Single Level 1 Attunement

- Part One – From the Back

The student's hands must be in "Namaste" position at the heart, eyes gently closed.

Draw the Fire Serpent from the crown to the root.

Draw Dai Ko Myo, Cho Ku Rei and Hon Sha Ze Sho Nen at the base of the spine.

Place both your hands on the student's head (link and ground).

Draw Dumo above the head (name x 3) and move through the crown to the base of the brain.

Draw Dai Ko Myo above the head (name x 3) and move through the crown to the base of the brain.

Touch the student's shoulder – Student to move their hands to the crown (holding "Namaste" position).

Draw Cho Ku Rei above the student's hands (name x 3) and move through the hands down to the crown and down to the base of the brain.

Move the student's hands back to the heart.

- Part Two – From the Front

Open the student's hands and cup the hands you're your non-dominant hand.

Draw Cho Ku Rei over the forehead (name x 3) and move through the head to the 3rd eye.

Draw Cho Ku Rei above the hands (name x 3) and move into the palms – tap x 3.

Place the student's hands back to "Namaste" position and "T" hands over – Blow over the hands down to the solar plexus and up to the 3rd eye and crown and then down to the hands.

- Part Three – From the Back

Place your hands on the student's shoulders – look down to the crown chakra and to the heart chakra.

Place affirmation into heart the chakra (x 3).

"You are a pure and divine channel of Reiki".

Place your hands together – thumbs at the base of the skull.

"I honour the love and light within you and am grateful to have shared this space in time, in touch, in love with you".

Visualize a door at the back of the head – Move Cho Ku Rei in and close and seal the door.

Place your hands on the student's shoulders and silently say this blessing - "We are both blessed by this process".

Disconnect from the energy with Raku.

Place the student's hands, palms up on the thighs, inhale slowly and gently open their eyes.

RM (Reiki Master) to re-centre.

Cho Ku Rei, Hon Sha Ze Sho Nen and Sei He Ki into the 3rd eye – Three separate attunements per symbol.

Cho Ku Rei - into the hands.

Combined Level 1 Attunement

- Part One – From the Back

The student's hands must be in "Namaste" position at the heart, eyes gently closed.

Draw the Fire Serpent from the crown to the root.

Draw Dai Ko Myo, Cho Ku Rei and Hon Sha Ze Sho Nen at the base of the spine (can tap it in x 3).

Place both your hands on the student's head (link and ground).

Draw Dumo above the head (name x 3) and move through the crown to the base of the brain.

Draw Dai Ko Myo above the head (name x 3) and move through the crown to the base of the brain.

Touch the student's shoulder – Student to move their hands to the crown (holding "Namaste" position).

Draw Cho Ku Rei above the student's hands (name x 3) and move through the hands down to the crown and down to the base of the brain.

Move the student's hands back to the heart.

Draw Sei He Ki and Hon Sha Ze Sho Nen above the head (name x 3) and move through the crown to the base of the brain.

Repeat steps 7 to 9 again – Cho Ku Rei into the hands.

- Part Two – From the Front

Open the student's hands and cup the hands with your non-dominant hand.

Draw Cho Ku Rei over the forehead (name x 3) and move through the head to the 3rd eye.

Draw Cho Ku Rei above the hands (name x 3) and move into the palms - tap x 6 (3 x on each hand).

Draw Sei He Ki and Hon Sha Ze Sho Nen over the forehead (name x 3) and move through the head to the 3rd eye.

Move the student's hands back to "Namaste" position and "T" hands over - Blow over the hands down to the solar plexus and up to the 3rd eye and crown and down to the hands.

- Part Three – From the Back

Place your hands on the student's shoulders - look down to the crown chakra and to the heart chakra.

Place affirmation into heart chakra (x 3).

"You are a pure and divine channel of Reiki".

Place your hands together with your thumbs at the base of the skull.

"I honour the love and light within you and am grateful to have shared this space in time, in touch, in love with you".

Visualize a door at the back of the head - Move Cho Ku Rei in and close and seal the door.

Place your hands on the student's shoulders and silently say this blessing - "We are both blessed by this process".

Disconnect from the energy with Raku.

Place the student's hands, palms up on the thighs, inhale slowly and gently open their eyes.

RM (Reiki Master) to re-centre.

Cho Ku Rei, Hon Sha Ze Sho Nen and Sei He Ki into the 3rd eye – One attunement.

Cho Ku Rei - into the hands.

Level 2 Attunement

- Part One – From the Back

The student's hands must be in "Namaste" position at the heart, eyes gently closed.

Draw the Fire Serpent from the crown to the root.

Draw Dai Ko Myo, Cho Ku Rei and Hon Sha Ze Sho Nen at the base of the spine.

Place both your hands on the student's head (link and ground).

Draw Dumo above the head (name x 3) and move through the crown to the base of the brain.

Draw Dai Ko Myo above the head (name x 3) and move through the crown to the base of the brain.

Touch the student's shoulder – Student to move their hands to the crown (holding "Namaste" position).

Draw Cho Ku Rei, Sei He Ki and Hon Sha Ze Sho Nen through the student's hands down to the crown and down to the base of the brain.

- Part Two – From the Front

Open the student's hands and cup the hands with your non-dominant hand.

Draw Cho Ku Rei, Sei He Ki and Hon Sha Ze Sho Nen over the forehead to the 3rd eye.

Draw Cho Ku Rei, Sei He Ki above the palms, tap x 3.

Place the student's hands back to "Namaste" position and "T" hands over – Blow over the hands down to the solar plexus and up to the 3rd eye and crown and then down to the hands.

- Part Three – From the Back

Place your hands on the student's shoulders – look down to the crown chakra and to the heart chakra.

Place affirmation into heart the chakra (x 3).

"You are a pure and divine channel of Reiki".

Place your hands together – thumbs at the base of the skull.

"I honour the love and light within you and am grateful to have shared this space in time, in touch, in love with you".

Visualize a door at the back of the head - Move Cho Ku Rei in and close and seal the door.

Place your hands on the student's shoulders and silently say this blessing - "We are both blessed by this process".

Disconnect from the energy with Raku.

Place the student's hands, palms up on the thighs, inhale slowly and gently open their eyes.

RM (Reiki Master) to re-centre.

All Usui symbols - into the hands.

Level Three Attunement

- Part One - From the Back

The student's hands must be in "Namaste" position at the heart, eyes gently closed.

Draw the Fire Serpent from the crown to the root.

Draw Dai Ko Myo, Cho Ku Rei and Hon Sha Ze Sho Nen at the base of the spine.

Place both your hands on the student's head (link and ground).

Touch the student's shoulder - Student to move their hands to the crown (holding "Namaste" position).

Draw Dumo above the hands (name x 3) and move through the hands to the crown and to the base of the brain.

Repeat with the Fire Serpent, Dai Ko Myo, Cho Ku Rei, Sei He Ki and Hon Sha Ze Sho Nen.

Move the student's hands back to the heart.

- Part Two – From the Front

Open the student's hands and cup the hands with your non-dominant hand.

Draw Dumo above the hands (name x 3) and move through the head to the 3rd eye.

Repeat with the Fire Serpent, Dai Ko Myo, Cho Ku Rei, Sei He Ki and Hon Sha Ze Sho Nen.

Draw Dumo above the hands (name x 3) and move into the palms, tap x 3.

Repeat all the above - above the hands (name x 3) and move into the palms, tap x 3.

Place the student's hands back to "Namaste" position and "T" hands over – Blow over the hands down to the solar plexus and up to the 3rd eye and crown and then down to the hands.

- Part Three – From the Back

Place your hands on the student's shoulders – look down to the crown chakra and to the heart chakra.

Place affirmation into heart the chakra (x 3).

"You are a pure and divine channel of Reiki".

Place your hands together – thumbs at the base of the skull.

"I honour the love and light within you and am grateful to have shared this space in time, in touch, in love with you".

Visualize a door at the back of the head – Move Cho Ku Rei in and close and seal the door.

Place your hands on the student's shoulders and silently say this blessing - "We are both blessed by this process".

Disconnect from the energy with Raku.

Place the student's hands, palms up on the thighs, inhale slowly and gently open their eyes.

RM (Reiki Master) to re-centre.

CHAPTER 4

Distant Attunement

The process of a Distant Attunement is very similar to that of a hands-on attunement and works on the same principles of distant healing.

As a Reiki Master, you may be required to perform a Distant Attunement for a student at some stage.

However, some Reiki Masters prefer to use this procedure for a Healing Attunement instead.

How to Perform a Distant Attunement

Set a time that is suitable for yourself and the student. You may undertake to do the attunement either telephonically, on-line or in absolute absence.

The student has to prepare approximately 20 minutes prior to the attunement, by praying, meditating or any activity which he or she would use to clear their mind.

Both the Reiki Master and student have to clearly state the intention of the attunement which is to take place.

Draw the distant symbol (Hon Sha Ze Sho Nen) in the air, with the intention that the attunement is to be fully empowering to the student and then begin the attunement process as normal.

You may also choose to undertake the attunement on a surrogate item, such as a teddy bear.

In order to fully allow the student to be attuned to Reiki, with this process, you need to ensure that you hold a clear and focused intention whilst doing this attunement.

Self-Attunements

Once you have been attuned, it will never fade or disappear. However, by doing a self-attunement, it will strengthen the reiki energy and the connection to source. These techniques are very powerful and this can be a wonderful spiritual experience.

You do not need a re-attunement, but all it will do is re-open up all the channels and strengthen the reiki energy. A self-attunement essentially offers you a boost. Many Reiki Masters choose to do a self-attunement on a weekly basis.

Therefore, you can do this once a week or whenever you feel like doing so.

Self-Attunement Using a Ki Ball

For this attunement, you will use the Level 3 attunement process.

Centre and ground yourself, as you would normally do.

Raise your arms above your head, with your palms facing upwards.

Visualize the reiki energy moving down your body, around your arms and surrounding you. Breathe in the energy and feel your palms soaking up the energy, entirely filling your being.

Lower your arms and put your hands in front of your chest, your palms approximately 2.5cm apart (facing each other).

Focus on the energy and allow your hands to slowly move apart. Visualize the energy between the palms, as a ball. Slowly grow the ball to the size of a soccer ball.

Perform the Master Attunement on the ball of Ki. "Imprint" the reiki symbols onto the ball.

Then draw the distant symbol (Hon Sha Ze Sho Nen) on the ball with the intention that this attunement should be sent to you.

Take a moment to receive the attunement.

Seal in the attunement, with your preferred method.

Return your hands to Gasshô and experience the energy for a while.

You may also choose to take the Ki ball and lift it above your head and drop the ball into your crown chakra, all the way down to the root chakra.

Let the ball bounce up and down and you will see the symbols bouncing off and going where they have to go.

It is important to relax a little longer after this process.

Alternatively, you may choose to use the surrogate process for the self-attunement. A good method to do this is to use the various areas on your legs to represent your body. As per the example below.

The right leg may represent the back of your body. The knee being the head and the thigh would be the length of the spine.

The left leg may represent the front of the body, just below the knee cap would be the third eye and the mid-thigh would be the heart.

Attune each hand with each other.

A Self-Attunement will not only strengthen the reiki energy and your connection to source, it will also leave you feeling rejuvenated.

IMAGE OBTAINED FROM PIXABAY (SEPTEMBER 2016)

CHAPTER 5

Advanced Reiki Techniques

In addition to the techniques you have been taught thus far, there are further advanced reiki techniques, which can be used in conjunction with a standard reiki session (on others) or on your students.

Psychic Surgery

Use the Term "Blockage Removal"

This can be done in conjunction with a standard reiki session, but the psychic surgery will be done first.

Centre and ground yourself and allow the client to prepare him or herself.

Ask the client to describe their concern. (What it is that they wish to have healed). You need to know the specific problem - what it is and where it is. It could be an emotional problem i.e. the loss of a child.

Ask the client to close his or her eyes and meditate on the issue. However, many people cannot meditate, so you need to ask the client to focus on the issue.

Ask the Client that if this was in the physical body, in which part would it be? This should be easy for the client, as one normally experiences tension or pain in a certain area, when you think of a certain issue.

If the client cannot pinpoint an exact area in the body, ask him or her to guess, suggesting that there is no wrong answer. Their instinct will be better than yours.

Teach your clients to trust their instinct.

Ask the client to imagine that he or she is looking into the area they have chosen and ask the client - if this was a shape, what shape would it be?

Ask the client to look into the chosen area, for this shape (which represents the negative energy which causes or signifies the issue).

It is important for the client to see the shape as negative energy, surrounding the organs or an area in the body, which has the problem, rather than looking at the shape of the physical organs.

This is vitally important, as you need to know exactly what you are going after and when to stop the "blockage removal".

Do the same with color, texture, weight and sound, in order that the client has a clear image of the "block". The client need to be clear about the blockage, but remember that any answer is acceptable, as the client does not have to get all of these things.

Tell the client that you will send the problem up to God, or "The Higher Power" or "The Divine Creator" and ask the client to meditate on releasing it.

Also ask the client to focus on the blockage (shape) and to observe any changes and to tell you about it. The client needs to be focused - constantly ask the client about the changes.

Also ask the client to be willing and open to receive and acknowledge any lesson(s) related to the healing process.

How to Perform Psychic Surgery
"Blockage Removal"

The client may stand or sit in a chair.

Stand behind the client. Draw the Usui master symbol (Dai Ko Myo) on both your hands and clap them together three times. (Repeating its name to yourself three times). Repeat this process with the power symbol (Cho Ku Rei). Then protect your energy by drawing the power symbol down the front of your body and over each chakra, to protect them.

Now you have to create "Reiki Fingers". You do this by "pulling" on your fingers and visualizing that they are extending by 15cm to 20cm. Then touch your imaginary fingers, imagining that you can feel them and draw the power symbol on the end of your fingers. You have to move your hands around and imagine that you can feel them and the power which they hold.

Do your opening prayer (silently or out loud). Call on your guides, angels, archangels and all healing beings of light, to assist you in creating the most powerful healing possible. Request that the healing should take place within divine love and for the greatest good of all concerned.

Draw the power symbol (Cho Ku Rei) on the client, over the area where the blockage is located.

With a powerful posture, use the full strength of your entire being and visualize reaching in and removing the blockage (negative energy) with your "Reiki Fingers". Visualize pulling it out and then flick this energy into the flame of a candle. (This sends it into the light, for transmutation). You have to do this procedure with spiritual, mental, emotional and physical intention. You may be able to feel or see the negative shape, or you may sense it in some way. Use your own insight to guide you in pulling this negative shape (energy) out.

Continue pulling this negative energy out for as long as you are guided to do so. You may experience a change in how the area feels and this means that you are making progress. Pull at this negative shape (energy) from different sides and/or angles. Allow your intuition to guide you through this process - how to do it and for how long to continue. However, do not rely on your instinct alone, the client has to be fully and actively engaged in this whole process.

Ask the Client to continuously give you feedback and if he or she is experiencing any changes in the shape of the negative energy. If there are no changes taking place, you may draw the mental/emotional symbol (Sei He Ki) on the area and hold your hands on it. Ask the area for guidance and whether there is a lesson to be learned, in order for the negative energy to be released. Also ask the client to focus on the area and to tell you whatever comes to mind. (Even if this seems irrational, crazy or embarrassing). By doing this, you are pushing it back into the client's consciousness, to see what the problem is and to deal with it.

Remain in your "zone" and stay focused on your client. Rely on your intuition and the guidance that comes to you. Sometime the issue can be resolved in one session, such as allowing love to enter in or to forgive someone for something. It may also happen that there could be a process which will have to continue after the session.

Continue pulling out the Shape (negative energy) after receiving and/or acting on the guidance that you have received and ask the client to give you feedback on the results.

Sometimes it is possible to release all the negative energy with one session, but it could also happen that a release process is initiated and may continue for several hours or days after the session.

After the session, you need to fill the area with reiki energy and seal the healing energy in with the power symbol (Cho Ku Rei).

Draw the Raku symbol in the air, between you and the client, in order to break the connection. Then retract your "Reiki Fingers", by pushing them back (imagining that they are returning back to normal).

You may then continue with a standard reiki treatment.

Additional Techniques and Exercises

Hatsurei Hô - Reiki Blessing

Mon Shisei - Standard Position

Sit in Gasshô and Seiza position (meditation position, with your legs crossed) with your eyes closed, to ground and centre your energy and to set the intention.

Then recite the five reiki precepts. (But this is not compulsory, it is optional).

Mokunen - Intention

Ground and centre your energy. Call in your guides and angles and set your intention.

Kenyoko Hô - Dry Bathing or Brushing Off

Stand in Gasshô position - ground and centre your energy and set the intention.

Arms at your sides - put your right hand on your left shoulder, with your fingertips touching the point where the collar-bone ends. Breathe in (through the nose) and as you breathe out intensely (through the mouth) move your hand diagonally across your body - from the left shoulder towards the right hip (use a smooth brushing action).

Arms at your sides - put your left hand on your right shoulder, with your fingertips touching the point where the collar-bone ends. Breathe in (through the nose) and as you breathe out intensely (through the mouth) move your hand diagonally across your body - from the right shoulder towards the left hip (use a smooth brushing action).

Lift your left arm (to form a straight horizontal line to the ground) palms facing down. Place your right hand on your left forearm. Breathe in (through the nose) and as you breathe out intensely (through the mouth) move your hand along the top of your left forearm sweeping all the way down over your fingertips.

Lift your right arm (to form a straight horizontal line to the ground) palms facing down. Place your left hand on your right forearm. Breathe in (through the nose) and as you breathe out intensely (through the mouth) move your hand along the top of your right forearm sweeping all the way down over your fingertips.

Return to Gasshô position and give thanks.

Jôshin Kokyû Hô - Cleansing Breathing

Sit comfortably and place your hands in your lap, with your palms facing upwards.

Breathe in deeply, through your nose and exhale through the mouth. Whilst you are breathing out visualize your energy expanding out of your body (through your skin) and into your immediate surroundings. When you breathe in, take energy in and when you breathe out, push the energy out.

Repeat the above two steps for as long as you are guided to do so. If you feel dizzy when doing this, stop the exercise. Over time and with practice, you will be able to do this for a longer period of time.

Seishin Toitsu - Concentration and Focus

In a standing position, place your hands in Gasshô position.

Focus on your hara line. Breathe in deeply through your nose and breathe out through the mouth. Whilst breathing in, bring the energy into your hands and feel the energy moving down your arms and through your body, into the hara.

Whilst breathing out, visualize the energy moving from the hara, back up into your body, through your arms and out through your hands.

Repeat the above two steps for as long as you are guided to do so. If you feel dizzy when doing this, stop the exercise. Over time and with practice, you will be able to do this for a longer period of time.

Recite the five reiki precepts. (But this is not compulsory, this is optional).

Return to Gasshô positions and give thanks.

The above exercise is very effective for the following:

- It boosts your energy.

- It opens the palm chakras, thus enhancing your ability to scan energy (prior to a treatment).

- It is very effective before doing a distant healing.

- This is also very effective prior to doing a manifestation.

CHAPTER 6

Reiju

You can do this exercise on anyone, but if you do this on someone who has never received a reiki treatment before, they have to keep their eyes closed.

Reiju is an empowerment procedure, which connects the student to the reiki source and strengthens the reiki connection. It enables a much deeper and stronger flow of the reiki energy. The student has the most important role in his or her own development.

Reiju enhances the reiki channel, but it is up to the student to further develop this channel, by continually practicing different techniques i.e. Hatsurei Hô (reiki blessing) and other additional techniques that we have covered so far.

The translation of Reiju, which is most commonly accepted, is "the giving of the five blessings". These five blessings are as follows:

1. The blessing of faith (confidence)

2. The blessing of zeal (energy and effort)
3. The blessing of mindfulness
4. The blessing of meditation
5. The blessing wisdom

Reiju allows for more Universal Life Force Energy to flow through the student and/or client, as it ultimately strengthens the connection to the reiki source.

It also helps to develop the one's intuition and sensitivity to energy. Receiving Reiju can benefit any practitioner on any level of reiki.

Building Your Energy Prior to Performing Reiju

If you are planning on doing multiple empowerments, you need to build reiki energy in your tanden. (You have to ensure to build your energy first, prior to doing any empowerments).

Lift your hands high above you, with your fingers splayed (your hand opened wide) and feel the reiki energy entering in and coming down into your hands.

Move your arms down and outward (in a circular motion) and then inward, until your hands are resting in front of the tanden. Rest your right hand in your left hand, with your thumbs touching. Then focus the energy into the tanden.

Whilst inhaling, change your hand positions. Now allow your index fingers and thumbs to touch. The rest of your fingers should be splayed (wide open) as in the symbol of the sun. Now push your hands outward and slowly raise them upward towards the crown. This action signifies the opening of all the chakras, to receive more energy.

When your hands reach your crown, release your hands - this is the top of the circle. Whilst exhaling, bring your arms down and outward (in a circular motion) and then inward, until your hands are resting in front of the tanden. Now alternate and rest your left hand in your right hand, with your thumbs touching. Then focus the energy into the tanden.

You may repeat the above steps two more times. Alternate the hands resting position at the tanden each time. Allow the reiki energy to build up in the tanden. You have to ensure that the energy builds in intensity.

Symbol of the Sun

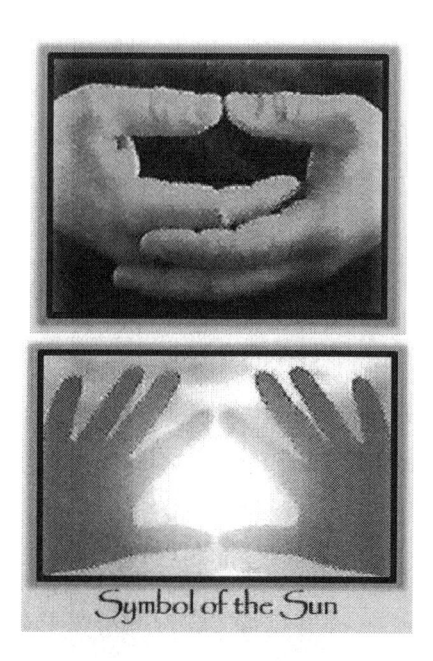

Giving a Reiju Empowerment

Allow the student and/or client to sit comfortably in a chair, with his or her hands in Gasshô position. Reiju is usually given in conjunction with the Hatsurei Hô sequence.

Stand in front of the student and/or client in Gasshô position and bow once.

Touch the student or client's shoulder to indicate that they have to put their hands together in Gasshô position (if they are not already in this position).

Lift your hands high above you, with your fingers splayed (your hand opened wide) and feel the reiki energy entering in and coming down into your hands.

The energy path: Move your hands down to just above the student or client's crown. Bring the first two joints of your index fingers together. You may relax your other fingers.

In one continuous motion, move your hands down in front of the student or client, drawing down a line of light, which enters the crown. Continue to trace an energy path down the centre of the body, with the intention that you are opening he energy centres, as you are doing so. Continue tracing this line, to the base of the spine. By now your hand will be close to the student or client's knees.

Separate our hands and with your palms facing down, move your hands sideways past the student or client's knees. Move your hands down towards the floor and ground the energy, but do not touch the floor. Then raise your arms outward and upwards, completing the circle above the crown.

Crown: With your palms facing down, move your hands down and touch the student or client's aura, just above their head, with your dominant hand and hold your non-dominant hand over the dominant hand. Now direct energy down the energy path, which you created with the previous hand movement. It is believed that this stage helps to "clear the energy body" and attune the energy body with the cosmic rhythm.

Temples: Move both your hands to both sides of the student or client's head, following the outline of the aura. Your palms should be facing the student or client's head (at the area of the eyebrows). It is believed by Hiroshi Doi that this expands the energy path and the student's entire body will be flooded with reiki.

Third eye: Following the outline of the aura, move your hands to the front of the student or client's face (with your palms facing the person's face) and make a triangle with your index fingers and thumbs (like the symbol of the sun). Hold the centre of this triangle in front of the student or client's third eye. Hiroshi Doi believes that this floods the third eye with light. It is said that this assist the third eye in functioning more sensitively and to connect with the higher consciousness. It enhances the intuition.

Throat: Hold one hand in front and one behind the throat and flood the throat with light. This is an intermediate step (not related to Hiroshi Doi).

Heart: Hold one hand in front and one behind the heart and flood the heart with light. This is an intermediate step (not related to Hiroshi Doi).

Hands: Allow the tips of your first three fingers to touch (the thumb, index finger and middle finger). Move your hands down and around the student or client's hands; but do not touch the person's hands. Allow energy to flow thought their hands and flood the hands with light. It is Hiroshi Doi's belief that the intention with this is to connect the "centre of the student" and "the centre of the universe". Now create an energy path from the shoulders to the arms, from the arms to the palms and integrate left and right energy.

For the above part of the process, the tips of your thumbs, index finger and middle fingers should be touching.

Release your hands in a smooth motion and move them downwards. Bring your hands together, before you reach the floor, palms facing upwards. Your little fingers should be touching (cup your hands) and your fingers should be pointed at the student or client. Move your hands up, towards the centre of the student or client's body, as if you are scooping the energy up and returning it to the sky. Move the energy along the energy path that you traced earlier. As your hands reach towards the sky, release your hands towards the end of this movement.

Return to Gasshô position and bow.

CHAPTER 7

Brain Balancing

This technique can be used to balance the left and right hemispheres of the brain. It is effective in the treatment of headaches, dyslexia and stabilizes epilepsy.

With this technique, energy is channelled in in one direction and the opposite. It can also be used on any part of the body, to remove energy blockages and to manage pain. This technique can balance both the client and practitioner.

The client can lay down or be comfortably seated in a chair. When you are using this technique on family or close friends, you may sit on the floor, with the person's head in your lap, as this is a very comfortable position.

This technique can also be incorporated into a standard reiki treatment. After conducting your interview with the client, you will know whether this technique may be required in the treatment session.

If the client has raised concerns such as headaches, anxiety, insomnia, or an inability to "switch off", then brain balancing is a good technique to incorporate into your treatment with the client.

Allow your intuition to guide you, it will never mislead you; you will know how to proceed...

How to do Brain Balancing

Stand in Gasshô position.

Centre and ground yourself, as you would normally do. Perform your opening procedure – opening prayer and connect to the earth's energy and allow the energy to run through your arms and hands.

Using two or three of your middle fingers, gently place your fingers on either side of the client's head, approximately 2cm above the ears. This is the area where there is an indentation, where the bones of the skull meet.

Channel energy from the one hand, through the brain and into the other hand. The other hand has to be receptive. Pay attention to the energy and/or any sensation of resistance that you may feel.

Continue to channel energy in one direction, until you feel it in the receptive hand. Then switch over and channel energy form the (previous receptive hand) in the opposite direction and into the other hand.

Continue to channel energy, changing direction when you feel the energy in the receptive hand and until there is an equal amount of resistance in both directions.

This technique takes approximately 3min to 5min and can be done every day or every second day.

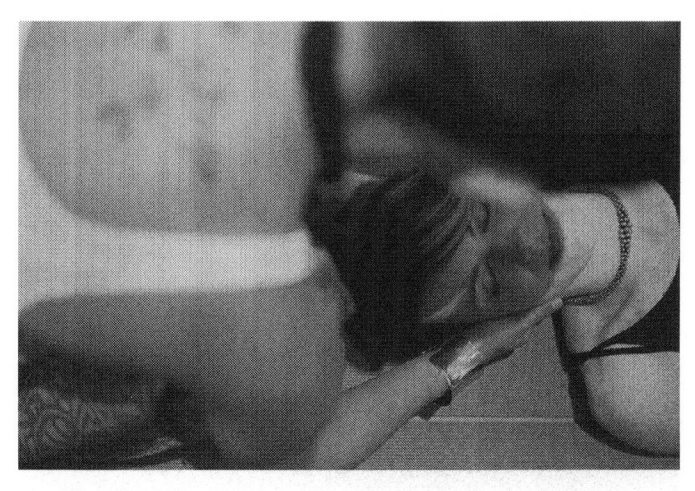

IMAGE OBTAINED FROM PIXABAY (SEPTEMBER 2016)

CHAPTER 8

Reiki Crystal Grids

A reiki crystal grid is an amazing technique to use for manifestation, protection and multiple distant healing.

You can charge clear quartz crystals with reiki energy. This charge will hold for approximately 48 hours and acts as a powerful link which transmits healing energy to you, your clients and your manifestations.

You will need the following:

6 x clear quarts terminators, of a similar size (single terminator).

1 x double clear quartz terminator.

1 x pyramid, cluster or sphere – use whichever setup or arrangement that you are guided to use.

Crystal cleansing methods:

Crystals can be cleansed by smudging them with incense.

You can soak them in salt water (in a glass bowl), which you may put in the sun or in the moonlight, overnight. It is important that you use tumbled crystals when you are using water to cleanse them.

You can also cleanse crystals by leaving them outside overnight, at full moon.

You can also cleanse crystals by leaving them overnight in brown rice (in a glass bowl). Ensure that the crystals are covered with the brown rice and discard the brown rice afterwards. (Do not use it).

Some practitioners also use Tibetan Singing Bowls to cleanse their crystals and/or Angel Cards.

Preparing your Reiki Crystal Grid

Cleanse all the crystals (use your preferred method).

Use the Symbol Meditation (used to focus and strengthen your channel). But, instead of raising the symbols down into the crown, you should visualize the symbols entering into the crystals. Ensure to only charge one crystal at a time.

Channel reiki into each crystal with the intention that they hold and transmit healing energy. Spend approximately ten minutes on each crystal. You can also do an attunement on each crystal.

Place the 6 x crystals (with an even distance between each crystal) on a circle - pointing inward. (Do not glue the crystals on the board).

Then place the pyramid or cluster in the centre of the circle. The six terminators all pointing to this crystal.

The double terminator acts as a charger or activator. In order to charge your grid, you will have to charge the double terminator with reiki energy every 48 hours.

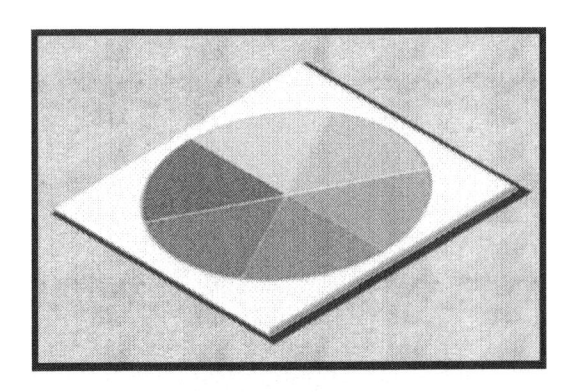

EXAMPLE OF A GRID

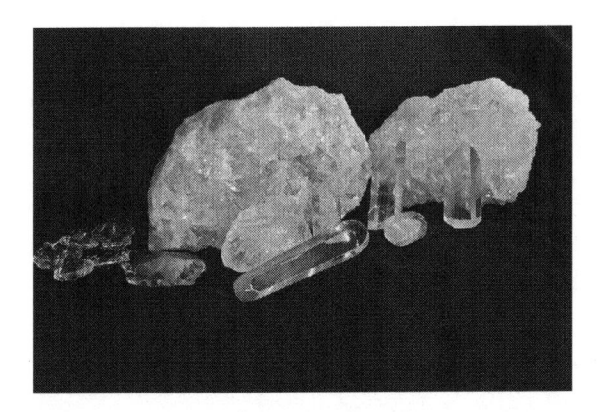

CLEAR QUARTZ - SINGLE AND DOUBLE TERMINATOR CRYSTALS

IMAGE OBTAINED FROM PIXABAY (OCTOBER 2016)

Charging the Grid

Once you have charged all the crystals, set your intention to charge the grid. Then trace out the pie shapes of your chart, from the central crystal to the end of each of the perimeter crystals (the 6 x outer crystals). This will process charge the grid.

"You were born with potential.
You were born with goodness and trust.
You were born with ideals and dreams.
You were born with greatness.
You were born with wings.
You are not meant for crawling, so don't.
You have wings.
Learn to use them and fly."
~ Rumi

CHAPTER 9

Teaching Reiki

Ethics

The practitioner's ethics which were covered in Usui Reiki Level 2 still very much remain part of a Reiki Master's journey, teachings and practice.

Bearing in mind the importance that reiki is energy, a Reiki Master who wishes to teach others should remain true to the spirit of reiki. You should strive to be a clear and true representation of reiki.

Teaching comes with both a blessing and a responsibility. As a teacher, you have a responsibility towards your students. That responsibility includes compassion, equality and respect.

You are blessed by being the one to open the door to reiki for your students, but you have to allow them to see what they will see.

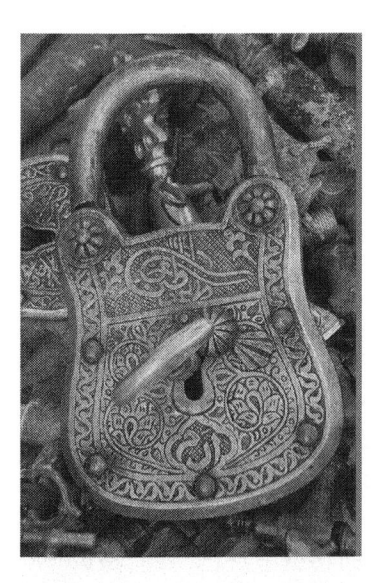

IMAGE OBTAINED FROM PIXABAY (OCTOBER 2016)

Preparing to Teach

Each Reiki Master has their own teaching style. But, we could easily fall into the habit of teaching others in the same way that we have been taught.

However, as we too learn and grow, we tend to change our teaching techniques to reflect our own level of personal understanding and our abilities.

As a teacher, you have to ensure that your teaching style is both comfortable and suitable to those who seek you out as a teacher. You also have to be willing to adapt your teaching style according to your students.

Be open-minded about teaching...

You may notice from time to time, how your teaching style varies, based on the students you are engaging with at any given time.

A good guideline would be to teach in such manner that you allow your students to also take the lead – let them explain how they understand the information you are providing them with.

It is important to be clear on what represents traditional Usui teachings and those techniques and practices which are non-traditional (modern-day) additions. You have to ensure that you cover the basic requirements of each level.

You have to ensure to teach your students the basics...

Points to Consider

Before you commit to facilitating a course, you need to consider a few important aspects, as follows:

- **Location**

You need premises where you can teach from and which can accommodate a few students at a time.

It is advisable not to enrol too many students at a time (many Reiki Masters choose to enrol only four or five students at a time).

You need to establish whether there is a demand for Reiki in your area.

If you do not have your own premises, it is important to consider the costs involved in renting premises.

- **Services/Facilities**

You need to consider whether you would like to offer refreshments i.e. coffee, tea or juice etc.

It is important to consider the costs involved in providing such facilities.

- Manuals and Certificates

You need to consider compiling and printing training manuals and Certificates.

You also need to consider whether you will conduct the printing yourself, or whether you will hire a professional to do so.

If you opt for hiring a professional, you need to consider the costs involved in the printing of your training material.

Teaching Aids

You need to consider which teaching aids you wish to include in your training course.

These normally include posters and cheat sheets etc.

Once again you would need to consider the printing of such materials and the cost involved in doing so.

- Course Dates and Timing

It is important to consider the date and time on which you wish to offer the training course.

You need to consider whether this will be a suitable date and time for prospective students.

It may be advisable to do some research first, prior to advertising and confirming your course date(s).

- Course Fees

After consideration of the above and establishing costs for printing etc. you may decide on the course fees.

It is important to ensure that your fees are neither too high nor too low. Therefore, it is recommended that you conduct some research on the fees that other Reiki Masters (in and/or around your area) are charging.

You may need to do some good old fashioned research and costing exercises before you just begin to teach.

Basic Class Outline - Reiki Level 1

The basic information that should be covered in a Reiki Level 1 course is as follows:

- What reiki is and how it works.
- The history of reiki.
- The five precepts of reiki.
- The standard reiki hand positions (for self-treatment and the positions for treatment on others).
- You have to demonstrate the hand positions and include enough time to practice the hand positions.
- Reiki Level 1 attunement.

Important Note

It is important to be clear on what represents traditional Usui teachings and those techniques and practices which are non-traditional (modern-day) additions.

You have to ensure to cover the basic requirements of each Module - Reiki Level 1 to Masters.

Optional Teachings

Apart from the standard minimum requirements and information which has to be covered, you may also include the following:

- o Additional meditation(s) and exercises. This may include effective grounding meditations and effective exercises to increase intuition and enhance a higher level of consciousness.

- o Additional Japanese techniques.

Basic Class Outline - Reiki Level 2

The basic information that should be covered in a Reiki Level 2 course is as follows:

- o What are reiki symbols.
- o Reiki symbol names.
- o Description and uses of the various reiki symbols.

- Drawing and activating the various reiki symbols

- You have to demonstrate the symbols and include enough time to practice drawing (and using) them.
- Reiki Level 2 attunement.

Optional Teachings

Apart from the standard minimum requirements and information which has to be covered, you may also include the following:

- Additional meditation(s) and exercises.

    This may include effective grounding meditations and effective exercises to increase intuition and enhance a higher level of consciousness.
- Additional Japanese techniques.

Basic Class Outline - Reiki Level 3

The basic information that should be covered in a Reiki Master (Level 3) course is as follows:

- The reiki master symbols.
- The names of the various master symbols.
- Description and uses of the symbols.
- Drawing and activating the various master symbols.
- You have to demonstrate the symbols and include enough time to practice drawing (and using) them.
- What it means to be a Reiki Master.
- Giving attunements.
- You have to demonstrate an attunement and include enough time to practice these techniques.
- Teaching reiki.
- Reiki Level 3 attunement.

Optional Teachings

Apart from the standard minimum requirements and information which has to be covered, you may also include the following:

- Additional meditation(s) and exercises.

   This may include effective grounding meditations and effective exercises to increase intuition and enhance a higher level of consciousness.

- Additional Japanese techniques.

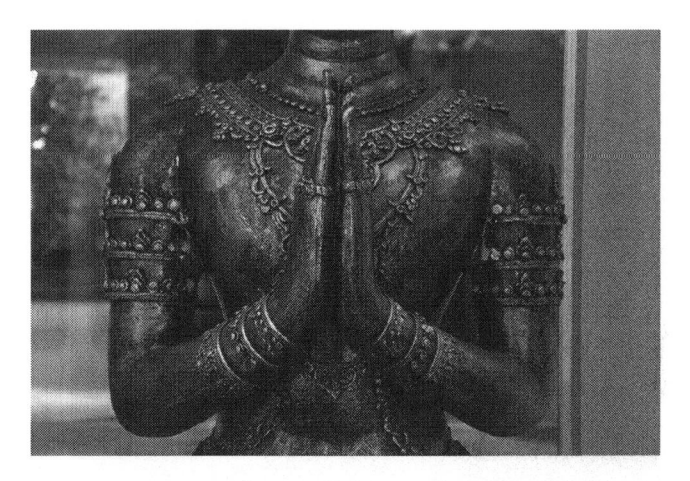

IMAGE OBTAINED FROM PIXABAY (OCTOBER 2016)

CHAPTER 10

Additional Techniques and Attunements

Non-Traditional

Microcosmic Orbit

This technique originated from Buddhist and Taoist meditative practices. It involves the conscious movement of energy through the main meridian system.

In this process you have to contract the Hui Yin and draw energy from the earth energies. Then place your tongue against the palate, just behind your teeth. This joins the conception (functional) and governing vessels and closes a full energy circuit along the Hara Line.

There are many Reiki Masters who teach this concept as a mandatory step, prior to passing the attunement to the student.

However, this is a rather advanced technique, which can take years to master. Therefore, many Reiki Masters do not consider this a mandatory step, to pass an attunement to a student.

Important Note

As this is not part of the original Usui Reiki teachings, it is highly recommended to research this technique more in depth, prior to commencing the practice thereof.

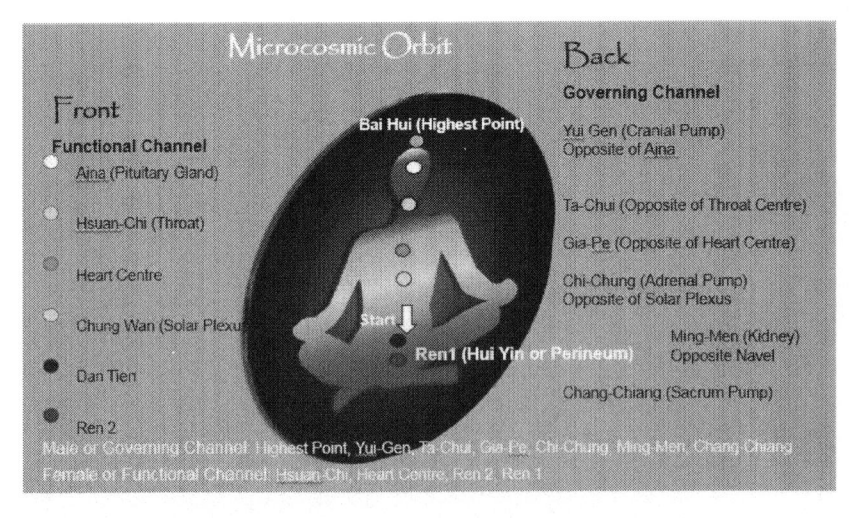

IMAGE OBTAINED FROM PIXABAY (OCTOBER 2016) AND EDITED/ENHANCED TO ILLUSTRATE "MICROCOSMIC ORBIT".

De-Attunement – Obedience Symbol

Praying against Reiki

This is a concept which is practiced mostly in European Countries. It is not a concept that is generally found within reiki circles in South Africa.

In the Usui Master Manual by Penny Jentoft, she explains in detail, the reasoning behind De-Attunements.

It does happen that some people change their minds about reiki, after already having undergone the reiki attunement process. They then go for what is called a "De-Attunement".

However, if one thinks of the principles of reiki and acknowledge the fact that reiki will always be with you; it will never fade and you can "never lose it". Then it is logical to assume that individuals who have been for a De-Attunement would be able to reactivate reiki at any time they wish to do so.

It is important that students should realize (prior to studying reiki) that being attuned to reiki is a permanent transformation. However, you also have the choice of practicing reiki or only studying reiki for your own personal improvement. (So, you are not in any way obliged to practice reiki).

It is said that that are some Reiki Masters in Europe, who have been using something called an "obedience symbol", which is used during the attunement process and binds the student to the Reiki Master. The student is then unable to use their own free will, to seek another teacher.

This is regarded as perverse abuse of the relationship between a Reiki Master and their student. Therefore, should you encounter someone who feels that they have fallen victim to this, you may assist them by treating this as if it were a blockage or deep seated emotional issue.

You would remove this by using the emotional/mental and empowerment healing techniques and further release this with affirmations. As reiki is self-protecting and works for the greater good of all, reiki cannot do any harm.

There are some individuals and groups who oppose reiki, based on their own personal, religious and spiritual beliefs and would pray to destroy reiki. Once could categorize this as some sort of psychic attack. But, no such cases have been reported where this practice has been successful.

The general idea seems to be that the people who oppose reiki are of the opinion that "anything that makes you feel good has to be bad".

The spirit of reiki acknowledges that "all is energy" and therefore the concept of De-Attunements and praying against reiki, is in direct conflict to the spirit of reiki.

These techniques are therefore considered misleading and as money-making rip-offs.

Reiki Assessments

When participating in the Reiki Master Level studies with a Reiki Master, you would be required to complete various assessments after receiving your Master Level Attunement.

These assessments are a valuable guide and measure as to the level of proficiency and knowledge that you have gained throughout your studies or Usui Reiki Healing.

You may expect and/or complete the following assessments:

- To give an appraisal (review) of your experience with the Hatsurei Hô Meditation (also known as a reiki blessing).
- To give an appraisal of your experience with Reiju (the empowerment process).
- To give an appraisal of your experiences with a healing attunement.
- To give a review of a self-treatment session, which had a particularly significant (meaningful) outcome for you.
- To provide two case studies of treatment sessions (of two different clients). Include information, such as their initial concerns, the treatment(s) given and techniques used. Also provide information on the outcome of these treatment sessions.
- To provide two case studies of distant healing sessions.

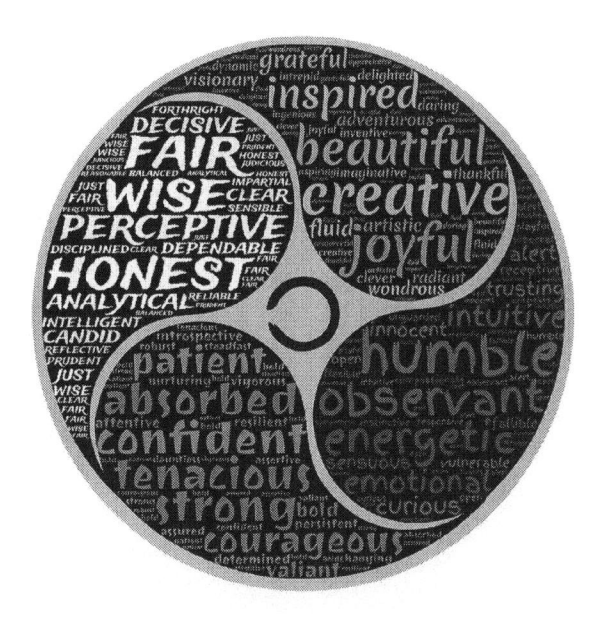

IMAGE OBTAINED FROM PIXABAY (OCTOBER 2016)

CHAPTER 11

ATTUNEMENT CHEAT SHEET

Single Level 1 Attunement

- Part 1 – From the Back

Students hands → Namaste @ heart, eyes closed

Fire Serpent ↓ crown to root

Draw DKM + CKR + HCZSN @ Base of spine

(RM) Both hands on client's head (link and ground)

DMO above head (name x 3) ↓ through crown to base of brain

DKM above head (name x 3) ↓ through crown to base of brain

Touch shoulder – student ↑ hands to crown

CKR above hands (name x 3) → through hands ↓ crown and ↓ to base of brain

Students hands ↓ back to heart

- Part 2 - From the Front

Open hands cup hands with non-dominant hand

CKR over forehead (name x 3) move through head to 3rd eye

CKR above hands (name x 3) move into palms - tap x 3

Student hands back to Namaste - blow over hands ↓ to solar plexus and ↑ to third eye and crown and ↓ to hands

- Part 3 - From the Back

Hands on shoulders - look ↓ crown chakra to heart chakra

Place affirmation into heart chakra (x 3)

"You are a pure and divine channel of Reiki"

Hands together - thumbs at base of skull

"I honour the light and love within you and am grateful to have shared this space in time, in touch, in love with you"

Visualise door at back of head - move CKR in and close & seal the door

Hands on shoulders - blessing "we are both blessed by this process"

Disconnect with RKU

Student palms up on thighs - inhale slowly - gently open eyes

RM re-centre

CKR / HSZSN / SHK into 3rd eye – three separate attunements per symbol

CKR into hands

Combined Level 1 Attunement

- Part 1 – From the Back

Students hands – Namaste @ heart, eyes closed

Fire Serpent ↓ crown to root

Draw DKM + CKR + HCZSN @ Base of spine (can tap it in)

(RM) Both hands on head (link and ground)

DMO above head (name x 3) ↓ through crown to base of brain

DKM above head (name x 3) ↓ through crown to base of brain

Touch shoulder – student ↑ hands to crown

CKR above hands (name x 3) move through hands ↓ crown and ↓ to base of brain

Students hands ↓ back to heart

SHK + HSZSN above head (name x 3) ↓ through crown to base of brain

Repeat steps 7 to 9 again (CKR into hands)

- Part 2 – From the Front

Open hands - cup with non-dominant hand

CKR over forehead (name x 3) through head to 3rd eye

CKR above hands (name x 3) move into palms – tap x 6 (3 x on each hand)

SHK + HSZSN over forehead (name x 3) through head to 3rd eye

Repeat Step 3 again (CKR into hands) It is not compulsory to repeat this step

Student hands back to Namaste – blow over hands ↓ to solar plexus and ↑ to third eye and crown and ↓ to hands

- Part 3 – From the Back

Hands on shoulders – look ↓ crown chakra to heart chakra

Place affirmation into heart chakra (x 3)

"You are a pure and divine channel of Reiki"

Hands together – thumbs at base of skull

"I honour the light and love within you and am grateful to have shared this space in time, in touch, in love with you"

Visualise door at back of head – move CKR in and close & seal the door

Hands on shoulders - blessing "we are both blessed by this process"

Disconnect with RKU

Student palms up on thighs - inhale slowly - gently open eyes

RM re-centre

CKR / HSZSN / SHK into 3rd eye – one attunement

CKR into hands

Level 2 Attunement

- Part 1 - From the Back

Students hands - Namaste @ heart, eyes closed

Fire Serpent ↓ crown to root

Draw DKM + CKR + HCZSN @ Base of spine (can tap it in)

(RM) Both hands on head (link and ground)

DMO above head (name x 3) → through crown to base of brain

DKM above head (name x 3) → through crown to base of brain

Touch shoulder - student move hands ↑ to crown

CKR + SHK + HSZSN through hands ↓ crown and ↓ to base of brain

- Part 2 - From the Front

Open hands - cup with non-dominant hand

CKR + SHK + HSZSN to → 3rd eye

CKR + SHK + HSZSN to palms - tap x 3

Student hands back to Namaste - blow over hands ↓ to solar plexus and ↑ to third eye and crown and ↓ to hands

- Part 3 – From the Back

Hands on shoulders – look ↓ crown chakra to heart chakra

Place affirmation into heart chakra (x 3)

"You are a pure and divine channel of Reiki"

Hands together - thumbs at base of skull

"I honour the light and love within you and am grateful to have shared this space in time, in touch, in love with you"

Visualise door at back of head – move CKR in and close & seal the door

Hands on shoulders - blessing "we are both blessed by this process"

Disconnect with RKU

Student palms up on thighs - inhale slowly - gently open eyes

RM re-centre

All USUI symbols into hands

Level 3 Attunement

- Part 1 – From the Back

Students hands – Namaste @ heart, eyes closed

Fire Serpent ↓ crown to root

Draw DKM + CKR + HCZSN @ Base of spine (can tap it in)

(RM) Both hands on head (link and ground)

Touch shoulder – student move hands ↑ to crown

DMO above head (name x 3) ↓ through crown to base of brain

Repeat with FIRE SERPENT/DKM/CKR/SHK & HSZSN

Students hands back to heart

- Part 2 – From the Front

Open hands - cup with non-dominant hand

DMO above hands (name x 3) through head to 3rd eye

Repeat with FIRE SERPENT/DKM/CKR/SHK & HSZSN

DMO above hands (name x 3) move into palms – tap x 3

Repeat ALL above hands (name x 3) move into palms – tap x 3

Student hands back to Namaste - blow over hands ↓ to solar plexus and ↑ to third eye and crown and ↓ to hands

- Part 3 – From the Back

Hands on shoulders – look ↓ crown chakra to heart chakra

Place affirmation into heart chakra (x 3)

"You are a pure and divine channel of Reiki"

Hands together – thumbs at base of skull

"I honour the light and love within you and am grateful to have shared this space in time, in touch, in love with you"

Visualise door at back of head – move CKR in and close & seal the door

Hands on shoulders - blessing "we are both blessed by this process"

Disconnect with RKU

Student palms up on thighs - inhale slowly - gently open eyes

RM re-centre

Healing Attunement

Begin the session as you would any "normal" session. Refer to your checklist (Usui Reiki Level 2 Manual).

Instead of laying down - client should be seated in an upright position (straight backed chair).

Ask the client the following questions:

Describe problem which he or she wishes to heal

If it were in the physical body - where would it be?

If it had a shape - what would it be?

If it had a color - what would it be?

Are you willing to release this blockage?

Ask the client to close their eyes - hands in their lap.

- Part 1 – From the Back

Fire Serpent ↓ crown to the root

Draw DKM + CKR + HSZSN @ Base of spine

(RM) Both hands on head (link and ground)

DMO above head (name x 3) ↓ through crown to base of brain

DKM above head (name x 3) ↓ through crown to back of heart

Repeat heart placement with CKR + SHK + HSZSN

- Part 2 – From the Front

DMO over crown (name x 3) → through 3rd eye ↓ to heart and ↓ to solar plexus

Gently tap crown with fingertips (x 3)

Repeat solar plexus placement with DKM + CKR + SHK + HSZSN

Gently blow ↓ toward solar plexus and ↑ toward 3rd eye and ↑ to crown and from the crown back ↓ to solar plexus (one fluid motion)

With intention (may use your hands to guide energy) on final sweep - ↑ upward to release negative energy and move it completely out of the energy system

- Part 3 – From the Back

(RM) hands on shoulders - visualize soft pink ball of energy at heart centre

Silently and lovingly repeat affirmation (x 3) - "You are empowered by love, light and wisdom".

Dominant hand on back of heart centre (other hand remains on shoulder). Affirm – "I now seal the healing process with love and light" or "I honour the light and love within you and am grateful to have shared this space in time, in touch, in love with you"

Return dominant hand to shoulder - silently say blessing - "We are both blessed by this process"

Disconnect with RKU

Move in front of client - have them place their palms on their legs, inhale and open their eyes on exhalation.

Ask client to concentrate on the negative shape and observe changes or its disappearance.

You may now proceed to do a "blockage removal" or a standard reiki session.

Conclusion

Firstly, congratulations on your decision to embark on this very meaningful journey of self-healing, growth, self-acceptance and self-love.

You have made a wise decision, which will not only better your life and offer you self-empowerment, but will change the lives of those who seek you out for healing or as a Reiki teacher.

Congratulations on successfully completing Usui Reiki Master Level training.

May your path be illuminated by love and light and may you be divinely guided as you move forward with the knowledge that you have acquired.

May you lovingly share this knowledge with those who seek your guidance…

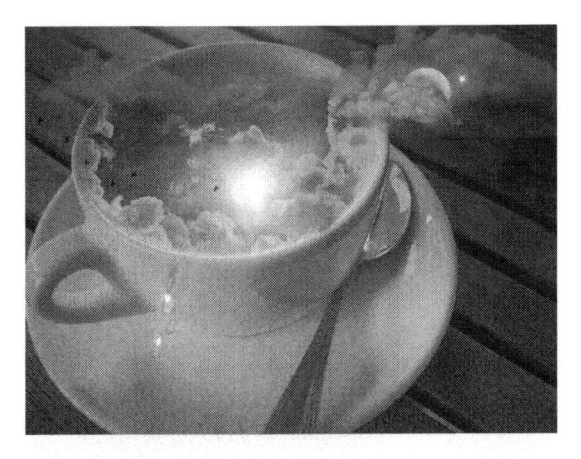

IMAGE OBTAINED FROM PIXABAY (OCTOBER 2016)

Final Thoughts

Always practice good Ethics.

As you gain experience, you may find and/or develop techniques which you may be more comfortable with; do not be afraid to use these techniques. Remember reiki energy will do what it is required to do.

Carefully consider the various points mentioned prior to facilitating any reiki courses.

Always remain true to the spirit of reiki.

Live by the five precepts. However, should you fail – try again tomorrow. Remember "For today only".

Always trust your intuition.

Always ensure that you intentions are pure.

Always ensure to practice "for the greater good of all concerned".

Always remember that each client will experience reiki differently – you cannot control the outcome.

Never omit to include a "Disclaimer" on your Client Information Form.

Remember that life is a journey – enjoy it!

Now that you have completed Reiki Master Level - Enjoy sharing your knowledge and insight with your students.

Those who require your unique gifts as a healer or teacher, will seek you out and their path will cross yours at just the right time... trust in divine timing...

I wish you much love and light on your journey!

Becoming a Reiki Master

Article by William Lee Rand

This article can be located on William Rand's website:

http://www.reiki.org/reikinews/reikin3.html

Reiki is a sacred practice that requires reverence and our greatest respect if we are to experience its most wonderful value. The benefits of Reiki can be all encompassing, not only giving us the ability to heal ourselves and others, which by itself is deeply meaningful, but also bringing guidance for our lives. Its unlimited nature can create opportunities for continual growth, unfoldment and the awakening of our own boundless potential.

The ever increasing joy, peace and abundance that await those who sincerely pursue the path of Reiki are not only a blessing to be enjoyed, but also contain the healing that the planet so dearly needs. Those who have been initiated into Reiki often feel this greater potential and aspire to continue on to the Advanced and Master levels. The desire to grow is inherent in simply being alive. As we look around ourselves and observe living things, we can clearly see that the one activity that all living things share is growth.

Everything that is alive grows. Because this is what living things do, one could even say that the purpose of life is to grow. Therefore, the desire to grow in ones Reiki potential is a natural expression of ones core essence and of life itself. If you feel this desire in your heart, honor and respect it. Doing so, will fulfil an innate need.

The joys of becoming a Reiki Master are many and you don't necessarily have to teach in order for the Master training to be useful. The additional healing energy, symbols, techniques and knowledge will add value to your healing abilities. Treating yourself, giving yourself and others healing attunements and treating others in person and at a distance will all be noticeably improved. The fact that you can pass Reiki on to friends and family is also a definite plus. Many take the Master training with just this in mind. However, if you ever decide to formally teach, you will be able to do so. As each person takes the Reiki Master training, and increases their personal vibration, this adds to the vibration of the whole planet!

One of the greatest joys of Reiki Mastership is teaching Reiki to others. Imagine the thrill of witnessing the members of your Reiki class receiving Reiki energy during the attunement. Then, as you guide them in its use, sharing in their joy and amazement as they experience its gentle power flowing through them for the first time. As your students use Reiki to help family, friends and clients, a wonderful sense of spiritual connection will develop between all of you. Feelings of compassion and love for everyone will be strengthened as you merge with the Reiki Consciousness and know more deeply that we come from God and that we are all one in God.

All information about Reiki has come to us through Mrs. Takata who learned the system of Reiki in Japan in 1935. According to Mrs. Takata, the definition of a Reiki Master is anyone who has received the Master attunement and Master symbol, understands how to give all the attunements and has actually taught a Reiki class thus passing Reiki on to others. Those who have taken Reiki Master training and not taught at least one person would not qualify as Reiki Masters and should call themselves Reiki Master Practitioners until they do teach. If you have taught a friend or family member, then you qualify as a Reiki Master.

After Mrs. Takata passed on in December, 1980, the twenty-two Masters she had initiated continued to teach and eventually began initiating other Masters. At first they taught in the same way Mrs. Takata had done, teaching the complete system in three degrees. Eventually some Masters began making changes to the system, adding knowledge and healing skills they had acquired from experience and inner guidance. Some took the third degree that originally contained the complete Master training and broke it up into two or more parts. Some actually broke the Master degree up into as many as five parts, calling each part a new degree.

When seeking a Reiki Master to take the Master training from, it is important to ask her/him exactly what you will be able to do after you take the Master training from them. Will you receive the complete training and be able to initiate others into all the degrees including full Reiki Master or will something be left out, requiring you to take additional sub-levels or degrees and pay additional fees?

Because of the changes some have made to the system of Reiki, this is a very important question.

Becoming a Reiki Master is a serious step that must be preceded by necessary preparation. One must first take Reiki I&II and Advanced Reiki training. It is also necessary to meditate on your life purpose and decide if Reiki Mastership is in harmony with it. Then, it is important to find a Reiki Master to study with who is competent and who you feel attuned to and will support you after you become a Reiki Master.

Becoming a Reiki Master implies that you will be able to initiate others into Reiki. Therefore, it is important to find a teacher who will spend time in class helping you practice the attunement process. Ask your teacher how much time is spent in class practicing the attunements as some teachers spend little or none.

Also ask them how much support they are willing to give you to begin teaching your own classes. This is important. Some Reiki Masters will have little interest in helping you get started as they are afraid you will take student away from them. If you are serious about becoming a successful teaching Reiki Master, find a teacher who will openly support you in achieving your goal.

Before teaching your first class, additional practice doing the attunements is a good idea. This can be done on friends who already have Reiki. Ask them if they would like to be an "attunement model" and let them know that the additional attunements will be beneficial for them and will refine and strengthen their Reiki energies. Most will gladly agree. If you can't find someone to practice on, you can use a teddy bear or a pillow to represent a person.

It will also be necessary to practice the talks, lectures and meditations you will be leading in class. Make outlines of your talks and practice into a tape recorder. Listen to your tapes and take notes on ways you can improve your talks. Then continue to practice until you are confident. Don't be afraid to use your outline in class. When teaching, relax and let the Reiki energy do the work.

If you have a sincere desire to help others and have taken the time to prepare to teach, you should have no trouble attracting students. It is your attitude that creates the results you receive so, assume success and you will create success. (See the previous two articles for ideas on promoting your practice)

As a teaching Reiki Master it is important to treat your students with the greatest respect. Know that each has the spark of God within them. Never use subtle threats or the withholding of information to cause your students to be dependent on you. Openly encourage each student to be connected to her/his own power and freedom of choice. What you create for others comes back to you. As you truly empower others, so will you be empowered. Trust in the abundance of the Universe and you will receive abundance and you will also be blessed with peace and joy.

When teaching Reiki to others, it is important to set a good example by being an authentic representative of Reiki energy. People cannot be so easily fooled by surface spirituality now. They want and need a real teacher who comes from experience and is working on her/his own deep healing. This requires one to meditate on the nature of Reiki energy and surrender to it. It is a continual process of working with all aspects of ones being that are out of step with Reiki energy and allowing those aspects to be healed by Reiki energy.

We must seek to develop and express the qualities of love, compassion, wisdom, justice, cooperation, humility, persistence, kindness, courage, strength, and abundance as Reiki energy is all of these and more. It may seem paradoxical, but it is true that a true Reiki Master is one who is always becoming a Reiki Master. Like life itself, it is a process of continual growth.

As you do this, you will realize sooner or later that there is more to Reiki than using it to heal yourself and others of specific problems. Reiki has a deeper purpose. In the same way that Reiki is able to guide healing energy when you are giving a treatment, Reiki can guide your life.

There is a perfect plan for your life that has always been present and has been waiting for you. This plan is exactly what is good and right and healthy for you. This plan is not based on what your parents want for you, or what the culture says you need to be accepted, but on what will really make you happy. This plan is inside you and comes from your core essence. Reiki can guide you to this plan and help you follow it. This plan is your true spiritual path.

By treating yourself and others and meditating on the essence of Reiki, you will be guided more and more by Reiki in making important decisions. Sometimes you will find yourself doing things that don't make sense or conform to what you think you should be doing and sometimes you will be guided to do things that you have vowed you would never do. However, by trusting more and more in the guidance of Reiki, by letting go of what your ego thinks it needs to be happy and by humbly surrendering to Reiki's loving power, you will find your life changing in ways that bring greater harmony and feelings of real happiness.

Over time, you will learn from experience that the guidance of Reiki is worthy of your trust. Once you have surrendered completely, you will have entered the Way of Reiki. When you do this, you will be at peace with the past and have complete faith in the future and know that there never was anything to worry about. Your life will work with ever greater harmony and you will feel that you have reached your goal of wholeness even as you continue to move toward it!

In the end, we must consider that a Reiki Master is not one who has mastered Reiki, but one who has been mastered by Reiki. This requires that we surrender completely to the spirit of Reiki, allowing it to guide every area of our lives and become our only focus and source of nurturing and sustenance. As we proceed toward the end of the millennium, the Way of Reiki offers itself as a solution to our problems and a path of unlimited potential. May all who would benefit from this path be guided to it.

Interesting References

Once you have completed Reiki Master Level, you have the option of continuing to practice reiki only, or you may choose to share your knowledge and insight with others and facilitate Reiki Courses.

As a Reiki Master, you should always remember that you have a responsibility to your students - respect, equality and compassion.

You have been blessed to be able to open the door to reiki for others, but allow them to see what they will see.

There are various books and resources available, not only in stores but also online, which offer further valuable insight and information about Reiki and energy.

Books Available Online

Below is a list of books you may find very resourceful.

The Essence of Reiki 3 - Usui Reiki Level 3 Master Teacher Manual: A step by step guide to the teachings and disciplines associated with Third Degree Usui Reiki

By Adele and Gary Malone

https://www.amazon.com/Essence-Reiki-teachings-disciplines-associated-ebook/dp/B0091UP2L2

The Reiki Sourcebook

By Bronwen and Frans Stiene

https://www.amazon.com/The-Reiki-Sourcebook-Bronwen-Stiene/dp/1903816556/ref=cm_lmf_tit_2

The Original Reiki Handbook of Dr. Mikao Usui

Dr. Mikao Usui and Frank Arjava Petter – Translated into English by Christine M. Grimm.

https://www.amazon.com/Original-Reiki-Handbook-Mikao-Usui/dp/0914955578/ref=pd_sim_14_3?ie=UTF8&psc=1&refRID=SXW4BHGN8Z0X43E4T2NW

The Japanese Art of Reiki: A Practical Guide to Self-Healing

By Bronwen and Frans Stiene

https://www.amazon.com/The-Japanese-Art-Reiki-Self-Healing/dp/1905047029/ref=cm_lmf_tit_1

Reiki The Ultimate Guide Learn Sacred Symbols & Attunements plus Reiki Secrets You Should Know

By Steve Murray

https://www.amazon.com/Ultimate-Sacred-Symbols-Attunements-Secrets/dp/0974256919/ref=pd_rhf_dp_s_cp_21?ie=UTF8&psc=1&refRID=TGQHFG31R65QBD3PDEV7

Reiki Master Manual: Including Advanced Reiki Training

By William Lee Rand

https://www.amazon.com/Reiki-Master-Manual-Including-Advanced/dp/1886785171

Additional Books on Reiki and Energy

The Spirit of Reiki

W. Lubeck, F. Arjava Petter & W. Rand

Hands of Light

Barbara Ann Brennan

Light Emerging

Barbara Ann Brennan

Wheels of Light

Rosalyn Bruyere

Interesting Reads to Guide You on Your Journey

In your quest to gaining further knowledge and attaining a higher level of spiritual growth, you may also find the following books to be insightful.

A Step in the Right Direction - Daily Devotional

Jennifer Rossouw

https://www.amazon.com/Step-Right-Direction-Daily-Devotional-ebook/dp/B00S2WGBLK

The Alchemist

Paulo Coelho

https://www.amazon.co.uk/Alchemist-Paulo-Coelho/dp/0061233846

The Teachings of Lao Tzu - The Tao Te Ching

Translated by Paul Carus

https://www.amazon.com/Teachings-Lao-Tzu-Tao-Te-Ching/dp/0312261098

Angel Therapy Handbook

Doreen Virtue Ph.D.

https://www.amazon.com/Angel-Therapy-Handbook-Doreen-Virtue/dp/1401918360

Sixth Sense

Stuart Wilde

https://www.amazon.com/Sixth-Sense-Stuart-Wilde-ebook/dp/B0043VDI7Y

The Crystal Bible 3

Judy Hall

https://www.amazon.com/Crystal-Bible-3-Judy-Hall/dp/1599636999

Your Body Speaks Your Mind

Deb Shapiro

https://www.amazon.com/Your-Body-Speaks-Mind-Understanding/dp/0749927836

Printed in Poland
by Amazon Fulfillment
Poland Sp. z o.o., Wrocław